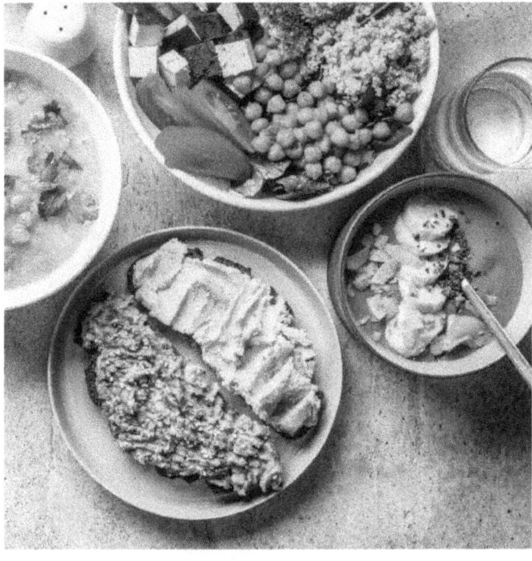

Nourish: A Culinary Odyssey through the Top 50 Superfoods for Vibrant Health"

Discover, Savor, Thrive – A Comprehensive Guide to Nutrient-Rich Foods and Their Transformative Impact on Your Body and Well-being"

Embark on a journey to vitality with "Nourish." Delve into the Top 50 Superfoods, where vibrant flavors meet health benefits. This culinary guide promises not just recipes but a transformative experience for your well-being. Ready to savor the extraordinary?

ZOHAIB HASSAN KHAN HEALTHY FOOD

Nourishing Every Home: A Guide to the Top 50 Most Healthy Foods"

AUTHOR

ZOHAIB HASSAN KHAN

This book provides comprehensive information on the top 50 most healthy foods, covering their uses, benefits, protein content, vitamin composition, calorie count, and their overall impact on the human body. Each chapter delves into the specifics of a particular food group, offering practical tips on incorporating these foods into everyday meals. With a focus on balanced nutrition, this guide serves as an invaluable resource for individuals seeking to enhance their well-being through mindful food choices.

1. Spinach

Uses:

Versatile ingredient in salads, sandwiches, and wraps.

Ideal for smoothies, soups, and sautés.

Can be used as a base for vegetable-based dishes.

Benefits:

Rich in iron, promoting healthy blood circulation.

Abundant in antioxidants, supporting overall health.

High fiber content aids digestion and promotes gut health.

Protein Content:

2.86 grams of protein per cup (cooked).

Vitamin Composition:

Excellent source of vitamins A, C, and K.

Contains folate, essential for cell division and DNA repair.

Provides a range of B-vitamins, contributing to energy metabolism.

Calorie Count:

Low-calorie option with approximately 7 calories per cup (raw).

Overall Impact on the Human Body:

Supports cardiovascular health and helps regulate blood pressure.

Contributes to bone health and reduces the risk of osteoporosis.

Aids in maintaining healthy skin and vision.

2. Kale

Uses:

Popular in salads, kale chips, and smoothies.

Adds a nutrient boost to soups, stews, and stir-fries.

Can be sautéed or baked for a crispy texture.

Benefits:

High in antioxidants, combating inflammation.

Loaded with vitamins, promoting overall immune health.

Supports detoxification with its sulfur-containing compounds.

Protein Content:

2.9 grams of protein per cup (chopped).

Vitamin Composition:

Rich in vitamins A, C, and K.

Contains significant amounts of manganese and copper.

Provides a good dose of vitamin B6.

Calorie Count:

Low in calories, with approximately 33 calories per cup
(chopped).

Overall Impact on the Human Body:

Aids in reducing the risk of chronic diseases.

Supports vision health and skin elasticity.

Contributes to the body's anti-inflammatory response.

3. Swiss Chard

Uses:

Great addition to salads, omelets, and sandwiches.

Suitable for sautéing, steaming, or braising as a side dish.

Can be used as a wrap for a nutrient-packed alternative.

Benefits:

High in antioxidants, protecting cells from damage.

Contains a variety of minerals essential for bone health.

Supports the body's natural detoxification processes.

Protein Content:

3.29 grams of protein per cup (cooked).

Vitamin Composition:

Excellent source of vitamins A, C, and K.

Rich in magnesium, potassium, and iron.

Provides a substantial amount of vitamin E.

Calorie Count:

Low-calorie choice, with approximately 35 calories per cup (cooked).

Overall Impact on the Human Body:

Supports cardiovascular health and helps regulate blood sugar.

Aids in digestion due to its fiber content.

Contributes to overall bone and immune system health.

4. Collard Greens

Uses:

Commonly used in Southern cuisine, often braised or stewed.

Ideal for wraps, especially when blanched briefly.

Can be added to soups, casseroles, and stir-fries.

Benefits:

High in antioxidants, combating oxidative stress.

Rich in vitamin K, essential for blood clotting.

Contains phytonutrients with anti-inflammatory properties.

Protein Content:

5.15 grams of protein per cup (cooked).

Vitamin Composition:

Exceptional source of vitamins A, C, and K.

Contains folate and choline, crucial for brain health.

Provides a range of B-vitamins, supporting energy metabolism.

Calorie Count:

Low in calories, with approximately 49 calories per cup (cooked).

Overall Impact on the Human Body:

Supports bone health and reduces the risk of fractures.

Contributes to a healthy immune system.

Aids in maintaining optimal cognitive function.

5. Arugula

Uses:

Adds a peppery flavor to salads, sandwiches, and pizzas.

Ideal for pesto, as a topping for bruschetta, or mixed into pasta.

Complements roasted vegetables and grilled meats.

Benefits:

14

High in nitrates, supporting cardiovascular health.

Rich in antioxidants, promoting overall well-being.

Contains compounds that may have anti-cancer properties.

Protein Content:

2.57 grams of protein per cup (raw).

Vitamin Composition:

Good source of vitamins A and K.

Contains significant amounts of folate and vitamin C.

Provides essential minerals such as calcium and potassium.

Calorie Count:

Low-calorie option, with approximately 5 calories per cup (raw).

Overall Impact on the Human Body:

Supports bone health with its vitamin K content.

Aids in maintaining healthy skin and vision.

Contributes to overall hydration due to its high water content.

6. Broccoli

Uses:

Versatile vegetable for stir-fries, salads, and soups.

Excellent when roasted, steamed, or blanched as a side dish.

Ideal for incorporating into casseroles and pasta dishes.

Benefits:

Rich in antioxidants, supporting overall health.

High in fiber, aiding digestion and promoting gut health.

Contains compounds with potential anti-cancer properties.

Protein Content:

2.82 grams of protein per cup (chopped).

Vitamin Composition:

Excellent source of vitamins C and K.

Contains folate, essential for cell division and DNA repair.

Provides a range of B-vitamins, supporting energy metabolism.

Calorie Count:

Low-calorie option, with approximately 31 calories per cup (chopped).

Overall Impact on the Human Body:

Supports cardiovascular health and helps regulate blood pressure.

Contributes to bone health and reduces the risk of osteoporosis.

Aids in maintaining healthy skin and vision.

7. Cauliflower

Uses:

Versatile ingredient for pizza crust, rice, and mashed potatoes.

Great when roasted, grilled, or added to casseroles.

Suitable for making soups, stews, and curries.

Benefits:

Rich in antioxidants, protecting cells from damage.

High in fiber, promoting digestive health.

Contains choline, essential for brain development and function.

Protein Content:

2.28 grams of protein per cup (chopped).

Vitamin Composition:

Good source of vitamins C and K.

Contains folate and vitamin B6, supporting brain health.

Provides essential minerals such as potassium and manganese.

Calorie Count:

Low-calorie choice, with approximately 27 calories per cup (chopped).

Overall Impact on the Human Body:

Supports detoxification processes in the body.

Aids in maintaining a healthy heart and reducing inflammation.

Contributes to overall well-being and immune system health.

8. Brussels Sprouts

Uses:

Excellent when roasted, sautéed, or added to salads.

Great as a side dish, especially when pan-fried or grilled.

Ideal for incorporating into stir-fries and pasta dishes.

Benefits:

High in antioxidants, combating inflammation.

Rich in fiber, promoting digestive health.

Contains glucosinolates, which may have anti-cancer properties.

Protein Content:

3.98 grams of protein per cup (cooked).

Vitamin Composition:

Excellent source of vitamins C and K.

Contains folate, supporting DNA synthesis and repair.

Provides essential minerals like manganese and potassium.

Calorie Count:

Low-calorie option, with approximately 56 calories per cup (cooked).

Overall Impact on the Human Body:

Supports bone health and may reduce the risk of fractures.

Aids in maintaining a healthy immune system.

Contributes to overall heart health and helps regulate blood sugar.

9. Cabbage

Uses:

Commonly used in coleslaw, stir-fries, and soups.

Ideal for fermenting into sauerkraut for probiotic benefits.

Suitable for stuffed cabbage rolls and casseroles.

Benefits:

High in antioxidants, protecting against chronic diseases.

Rich in fiber, promoting digestive health.

Contains glucosinolates, which may have anti-cancer properties.

Protein Content:

1.28 grams of protein per cup (shredded).

Vitamin Composition:

Good source of vitamins C and K.

Contains folate and vitamin B6, supporting overall health.

Provides essential minerals such as manganese and potassium.

Calorie Count:

Low-calorie choice, with approximately 22 calories per cup (shredded).

Overall Impact on the Human Body:

Supports detoxification processes in the body.

Aids in maintaining a healthy heart and reducing inflammation.

Contributes to overall well-being and immune system health.

10. Bok Choy

Uses:

Commonly used in Asian cuisine, stir-fries, and soups.

Great when sautéed, steamed, or added to noodle dishes.

Suitable for raw consumption in salads or as a crunchy snack.

Benefits:

High in antioxidants, protecting against oxidative stress.

Rich in vitamins A and C, supporting immune health.

Contains calcium and vitamin K for bone health.

Protein Content:

1.53 grams of protein per cup (shredded).

Vitamin Composition:

Excellent source of vitamins A and C.

Contains folate, supporting DNA synthesis and repair.

Provides essential minerals such as calcium and potassium.

Calorie Count:

Low-calorie option, with approximately 9 calories per cup (shredded).

Overall Impact on the Human Body:

Supports bone health and reduces the risk of osteoporosis.

Aids in maintaining a healthy heart and regulating blood pressure.

Contributes to overall well-being and may have anti-inflammatory properties.

Chapter 3: Berries

11. Blueberries

Uses:

Perfect for snacks, smoothies, and yogurt toppings.

Ideal for desserts, such as pies, tarts, and parfaits.

Incorporate into salads for a burst of sweetness.

Benefits:

High in antioxidants, supporting brain health.

Rich in fiber, promoting digestive health.

Contains anthocyanins, which may have anti-inflammatory properties.

Protein Content:

0.74 grams of protein per cup.

Vitamin Composition:

Excellent source of vitamin C.

Contains vitamin K, manganese, and a variety of B-vitamins.

Provides essential minerals like potassium.

Calorie Count:

Low-calorie option, with approximately 84 calories per cup.

Overall Impact on the Human Body:

Supports cognitive function and may reduce age-related decline.

Aids in maintaining healthy skin and vision.

Contributes to overall cardiovascular health.

12. Strawberries

Uses:

Excellent for fresh consumption and as a topping for cereals.

Great in smoothies, salads, and desserts.

Can be used in jams, jellies, and homemade sauces.

Benefits:

High in antioxidants, supporting heart health.

Rich in vitamin C, promoting immune function.

Contains ellagic acid, which may have anti-cancer properties.

Protein Content:

1.11 grams of protein per cup.

Vitamin Composition:

Excellent source of vitamin C.

Contains manganese, folate, and potassium.

Provides a range of B-vitamins.

Calorie Count:

Low-calorie choice, with approximately 50 calories per cup.

Overall Impact on the Human Body:

Supports cardiovascular health and helps regulate blood sugar.

Aids in reducing inflammation and promoting overall well-being.

Contributes to skin health and may have anti-aging effects.

13. Raspberries

Uses:

Perfect for snacks, breakfast bowls, and desserts.

Ideal for jams, jellies, and fruit sauces.

Incorporate into salads or as a topping for pancakes.

Benefits:

High in antioxidants, supporting overall health.

Rich in fiber, promoting digestive health.

Contains quercetin, which may have anti-inflammatory properties.

Protein Content:

1.48 grams of protein per cup.

Vitamin Composition:

Good source of vitamin C.

Contains manganese, folate, and potassium.

Provides essential minerals like copper.

Calorie Count:

Low-calorie option, with approximately 64 calories per cup.

Overall Impact on the Human Body:

Supports cardiovascular health and helps regulate blood pressure.

Aids in reducing inflammation and promoting overall well-being.

Contributes to skin health and may have anti-aging effects.

14. Blackberries

Uses:

Great for snacking, adding to salads, or topping desserts.

Ideal for smoothies, jams, and cobblers.

Incorporate into yogurt or as a complement to cheese plates.

Benefits:

High in antioxidants, supporting overall health.

Rich in fiber, promoting digestive health.

Contains anthocyanins, which may have anti-inflammatory properties.

Protein Content:

2.00 grams of protein per cup.

Vitamin Composition:

Good source of vitamin C.

Contains vitamin K, manganese, and folate.

Provides essential minerals like copper.

Calorie Count:

Low-calorie choice, with approximately 62 calories per cup.

Overall Impact on the Human Body:

Supports cardiovascular health and helps regulate blood sugar.

Aids in reducing inflammation and promoting overall well-being.

Contributes to skin health and may have anti-aging effects.

15. Cranberries

Uses:

Commonly used in sauces, juices, and baked goods.

Ideal for adding to salads or trail mixes.

Can be incorporated into stuffing or enjoyed as a dried snack.

Benefits:

High in antioxidants, supporting urinary tract health.

Rich in vitamin C, promoting immune function.

Contains proanthocyanidins, which may have anti-inflammatory properties.

Protein Content:

0.39 grams of protein per cup (whole).

Vitamin Composition:

Good source of vitamin C.

Contains vitamin E, K, and a variety of B-vitamins.

Provides essential minerals like manganese.

Calorie Count:

Low-calorie option, with approximately 51 calories per cup (whole).

Overall Impact on the Human Body:

Supports urinary tract health and may prevent infections.

Aids in reducing inflammation and promoting overall well-being.

Contributes to cardiovascular health and helps regulate blood pressure.

Chapter 4: Nuts and Seeds

16. Almonds

Uses:

A nutritious snack on its own or mixed with dried fruits.

Ideal as a topping for yogurt, oatmeal, or salads.

Used in baking, almond butter, and almond milk.

Benefits:

High in monounsaturated fats, promoting heart health.

Rich in vitamin E, an antioxidant for skin health.

Contains magnesium and phosphorus for bone health.

Protein Content:

6.02 grams of protein per ounce (approximately 23 almonds).

Vitamin Composition:

Good source of vitamin E.

Contains riboflavin, niacin, and folate.

Provides essential minerals like calcium and iron.

Calorie Count:

Moderate calorie option, with approximately 160 calories per ounce.

Overall Impact on the Human Body:

Supports heart health by reducing bad cholesterol levels.

Aids in maintaining healthy skin and preventing oxidative stress.

Contributes to bone health and energy metabolism.

17. Walnuts

Uses:

Excellent as a standalone snack or mixed with dried fruits.

Adds a crunchy texture to salads, oatmeal, or yogurt.

Incorporate into baking, smoothies, or as a nut butter.

Benefits:

High in omega-3 fatty acids, supporting heart health.

Rich in antioxidants, promoting overall well-being.

Contains melatonin, aiding in sleep regulation.

Protein Content:

4.32 grams of protein per ounce.

Vitamin Composition:

Good source of vitamin E.

Contains B-vitamins like folate and vitamin B6.

Provides essential minerals like copper and manganese.

Calorie Count:

Moderate calorie option, with approximately 185 calories per ounce.

Overall Impact on the Human Body:

Supports heart health by reducing inflammation and improving cholesterol.

Aids in reducing oxidative stress and inflammation.

Contributes to overall cognitive function and may improve sleep quality.

18. Chia Seeds

Uses:

Creates a gel-like texture when mixed with liquids, ideal for puddings.

Sprinkle on yogurt, oatmeal, or salads for added texture.

Incorporate into smoothies, baked goods, or as an egg substitute.

Benefits:

High in omega-3 fatty acids, supporting heart health.

Rich in fiber, promoting digestive health and satiety.

Contains antioxidants, reducing oxidative stress.

Protein Content:

4.69 grams of protein per ounce.

Vitamin Composition:

Good source of vitamins A and K.

Contains B-vitamins like niacin and riboflavin.

Provides essential minerals like calcium and phosphorus.

Calorie Count:

Moderate calorie option, with approximately 138 calories per ounce.

Overall Impact on the Human Body:

Supports heart health by reducing inflammation and improving cholesterol.

Aids in maintaining digestive health and regulating blood sugar.

Contributes to bone health and overall well-being.

19. Flaxseeds

Uses:

Ground flaxseeds can be added to smoothies, yogurt, or oatmeal.

Use as an egg substitute in baking.

Incorporate into salads, soups, or as a topping for casseroles.

Benefits:

High in omega-3 fatty acids, supporting heart health.

Rich in fiber, promoting digestive health.

Contains lignans, which may have anti-cancer properties.

Protein Content:

5.18 grams of protein per ounce.

Vitamin Composition:

Good source of vitamins B1, B6, and folate.

Contains vitamin E and K.

Provides essential minerals like magnesium and phosphorus.

Calorie Count:

Moderate calorie option, with approximately 150 calories per ounce.

Overall Impact on the Human Body:

Supports heart health by reducing inflammation and improving cholesterol.

Aids in maintaining digestive health and regulating blood sugar.

Contributes to bone health and may have anti-cancer properties.

20. Pumpkin Seeds

Uses:

Roasted pumpkin seeds make a nutritious snack.

Add to salads, yogurt, or oatmeal for a crunchy texture.

Incorporate into baked goods or use as a topping for soups.

Benefits:

Rich in magnesium, promoting heart health.

High in zinc, supporting immune function.

Contains antioxidants, reducing oxidative stress.

Protein Content:

7.05 grams of protein per ounce.

Vitamin Composition:

Good source of vitamins A, B2, B3, and B5.

Contains vitamin E and folate.

Provides essential minerals like iron and zinc.

Calorie Count:

Moderate calorie option, with approximately 151 calories per ounce.

Overall Impact on the Human Body:

Supports heart health by regulating blood pressure and cholesterol.

Aids in maintaining immune function and reducing inflammation.

Contributes to bone health and overall well-being.

Chapter 5: Whole Grains

21. Quinoa

Uses:

- Serves as a versatile base for salads, bowls, and side dishes.

- Can be used in place of rice or pasta in various recipes.

- Incorporate into breakfast dishes, such as porridge or granola.

Benefits:

- Complete protein source, containing all essential amino acids.

- High in fiber, promoting digestive health.

- Rich in antioxidants, supporting overall well-being.

Protein **Content:**

- 8.14 grams of protein per cup (cooked).

Vitamin Composition:

- Good source of vitamins B1, B2, B6, and folate.

- Contains vitamin E and minerals like iron and magnesium.

- Provides essential amino acids, supporting muscle health.

Calorie Count:

- Moderate calorie option, with approximately 222 calories per cup (cooked).

Overall Impact on the Human Body:

- Supports muscle growth and repair with its complete protein profile.

- Aids in maintaining digestive health and regulating blood sugar.

- Contributes to overall well-being with its rich nutrient content.

---

22. Brown Rice

Uses:

- A staple in various cuisines, serving as a side dish or base for meals.

- Ideal for stir-fries, casseroles, and stuffed peppers.

- Can be used in desserts, such as rice pudding.

Benefits:

- Rich in fiber, promoting digestive health.

- Contains selenium, supporting thyroid function.

- Provides sustained energy due to its complex carbohydrates.

Protein Content:

- 5.03 grams of protein per cup (cooked).

Vitamin Composition:

- Good source of vitamins B1, B3, and B6.

- Contains minerals like magnesium, phosphorus, and manganese.

- Provides essential amino acids, supporting muscle health.

Calorie Count:

- Moderate calorie option, with approximately 218 calories per cup (cooked).

Overall Impact on the Human Body:

- Supports digestive health and may aid in weight management.

- Contributes to thyroid function with its selenium content.

- Provides a steady release of energy and supports muscle health.

---

23. Oats

Uses:

- Commonly used for breakfast as oatmeal or overnight oats.

- Incorporate into baking, such as cookies, muffins, and granola.

- Can be used as a base for savory dishes, like oat-crusted chicken.

Benefits:

- High in soluble fiber, promoting heart health.

- Contains beta-glucans, supporting immune function.

- Rich in antioxidants, reducing oxidative stress.

Protein Content:

- 6.09 grams of protein per cup (cooked).

Vitamin Composition:

- Good source of vitamins B1, B5, and folate.

- Contains minerals like iron, magnesium, and zinc.

- Provides sustained energy due to its complex carbohydrates.

Calorie Count:

- Moderate calorie option, with approximately 154 calories per cup (cooked).

Overall Impact on the Human Body:

- Supports heart health and helps regulate cholesterol levels.

- Aids in maintaining immune function and reducing inflammation.

- Provides sustained energy and supports overall well-being.

---

24. Barley

Uses:

- Used in soups, stews, and risottos for a chewy texture.

- Can be used as a side dish, pilaf, or in salads.

- Incorporate into baked goods, like barley bread or muffins.

Benefits:

- High in fiber, promoting digestive health.

- Contains beta-glucans, supporting heart health.

- Rich in antioxidants, reducing oxidative stress.

Protein Content:

- 3.55 grams of protein per cup (cooked).

Vitamin Composition:

- Good source of vitamins B1, B3, and B6.

- Contains minerals like iron, magnesium, and phosphorus.

- Provides sustained energy due to its complex carbohydrates.

Calorie Count:

- Moderate calorie option, with approximately 193 calories per cup (cooked).

Overall Impact on the Human Body:

- Supports digestive health and may aid in weight management.

- Contributes to heart health and helps regulate blood sugar.

- Provides sustained energy and supports overall well-being.

---

25. Farro

Uses:

- Serves as a nutty and chewy base for salads and grain bowls.

- Ideal for soups, risottos, and pilafs.

- Can be used in breakfast dishes, like farro porridge.

Benefits:

- High in fiber, promoting digestive health.

- Contains antioxidants, reducing oxidative stress.

- Rich in nutrients like magnesium, iron, and zinc.

Protein Content:

- 7.03 grams of protein per cup (cooked).

Vitamin Composition:

- Good source of vitamins B1, B2, B3, and B6.

- Contains minerals like magnesium, iron, and zinc.

- Provides sustained energy due to its complex carbohydrates.

Calorie Count:

- Moderate calorie option, with approximately 220 calories per cup (cooked).

Overall Impact on the Human Body:

- Supports digestive health and may aid in weight management.

- Contributes to overall well-being with its rich nutrient content.

- Provides sustained energy and supports muscle health.

Chapter 6: Fruits

26. Apples

Uses:

A portable and convenient snack on its own.

Sliced apples make a healthy addition to salads and cheese plates.

Used in baking, such as pies, crisps, and muffins.

Benefits:

High in fiber, promoting digestive health.

Contains antioxidants, reducing oxidative stress.

Provides natural sweetness with a low calorie count.

Protein Content:

0.47 grams of protein per medium-sized apple.

Vitamin Composition:

Good source of vitamin C.

Contains B-vitamins like riboflavin and vitamin B6.

Provides essential minerals like potassium.

Calorie Count:

Low-calorie option, with approximately 95 calories per medium-sized apple.

Overall Impact on the Human Body:

Supports digestive health and may aid in weight management.

Contributes to heart health and helps regulate blood sugar.

Provides essential nutrients and antioxidants for overall well-being.

27. Oranges

Uses:

Juiced for a refreshing drink or as a citrusy addition to cocktails.

Sliced oranges make a healthy snack or topping for yogurt.

Used in salads, salsas, and desserts for a burst of flavor.

Benefits:

High in vitamin C, supporting immune function.

Contains antioxidants, reducing oxidative stress.

Provides natural sweetness with a low calorie count.

Protein Content:

1.23 grams of protein per medium-sized orange.

Vitamin Composition:

Excellent source of vitamin C.

Contains B-vitamins like thiamine and folate.

Provides essential minerals like potassium.

Calorie Count:

Low-calorie option, with approximately 62 calories per medium-**sized orange.**

Overall Impact on the Human Body:

Supports immune function and overall well-being.

Contributes to heart health and helps regulate blood pressure.

Provides hydration and essential nutrients with low calories.

28. Bananas

Uses:

A convenient and portable snack on its own.

Sliced bananas make a healthy topping for cereal, yogurt, or **pancakes.**

Used in smoothies, baked goods, and desserts for natural sweetness.

Benefits:

High in potassium, supporting heart health.

Contains vitamin B6, essential for brain development and function.

Provides natural sweetness with a moderate calorie count.

Protein Content:

1.29 grams of protein per medium-sized banana.

Vitamin Composition:

Contains vitamin C and B-vitamins like B6 and folate.

Provides essential minerals like potassium and magnesium.

Calorie Count:

Moderate calorie option, with approximately 105 calories per medium-sized banana.

Overall Impact on the Human Body:

Supports heart health and helps regulate blood pressure.

Contributes to brain health and overall well-being.

Provides a quick source of energy with natural sugars.

29. Avocado

Uses:

Sliced avocado is a creamy addition to salads, sandwiches, and wraps.

Mashed avocado is used as a spread, dip, or base for sauces.

Added to smoothies, desserts, and as a topping for toast.

Benefits:

High in monounsaturated fats, promoting heart health.

Contains fiber, promoting digestive health.

Rich in vitamins, including vitamin K, vitamin E, and B-vitamins.

Protein Content:

2.87 grams of protein per cup (sliced).

Vitamin Composition:

Excellent source of vitamin K.

Contains vitamins E, C, and a variety of B-vitamins.

Provides essential minerals like potassium and magnesium.

Calorie Count:

Moderate calorie option, with approximately 234 calories per cup (sliced).

Overall Impact on the Human Body:

Supports heart health and helps regulate cholesterol levels.

Aids in maintaining digestive health and promoting satiety.

Contributes to overall well-being with its rich nutrient content.

30. Papaya

Uses:

Sliced papaya is a tropical addition to fruit salads and desserts.

Blended into smoothies or juices for a refreshing drink.

Used in salsas, chutneys, and sauces for a sweet and tangy flavor.

Benefits:

High in vitamin C, supporting immune function.

Contains enzymes like papain, aiding in digestion.

Rich in antioxidants, reducing oxidative stress.

Protein Content:

1.10 grams of protein per cup (cubed).

Vitamin Composition:

Excellent source of vitamin C.

Contains vitamin A, E, and a variety of B-vitamins.

Provides essential minerals like potassium and magnesium.

Calorie Count:

Low-calorie option, with approximately 59 calories per cup (cubed).

Overall Impact on the Human Body:

Supports immune function and overall well-being.

Aids in digestion and may alleviate symptoms of digestive disorders.

Contributes to skin health and may have anti-inflammatory effects.

Chapter 7: Lean Proteins

31. Chicken Breast

Uses:

Grilled, baked, or sautéed for main dishes.

Sliced or shredded in salads, wraps, and sandwiches.

Added to soups, stews, and casseroles for protein.

Benefits:

High-quality protein for muscle maintenance and growth.

Low in saturated fats, promoting heart health.

Contains essential amino acids for overall well-being.

Protein Content:

Approximately 31 grams of protein per 3.5 ounces (cooked).

Vitamin Composition:

Contains B-vitamins like niacin and B6.

Provides essential minerals like phosphorus and selenium.

Low in calories, supporting weight management.

Calorie Count:

Lean option with approximately 165 calories per 3.5 ounces (cooked).

Overall Impact on the Human Body:

Supports muscle health and aids in weight management.

Contributes to heart health by being a lean protein source.

Provides essential nutrients for overall well-being.

32. Salmon

Uses:

Grilled, baked, or broiled for a flavorful main dish.

Added to salads, pasta, or rice dishes.

A rich source of omega-3 fatty acids for heart health.

Benefits:

High in omega-3 fatty acids, promoting heart health.

Rich in protein and essential amino acids.

Contains vitamin D for bone health and immune support.

Protein Content:

Approximately 25 grams of protein per 3.5 ounces (cooked).

Vitamin Composition:

Excellent source of vitamin D.

Contains B-vitamins like niacin, B6, and B12.

Provides essential minerals like selenium and iodine.

Calorie Count:

Nutrient-dense option with approximately 206 calories per 3.5 ounces (cooked).

Overall Impact on the Human Body:

Supports heart health and helps regulate cholesterol levels.

Contributes to bone health and immune function.

Provides high-quality protein for muscle maintenance.

33. Tofu

Uses:

Versatile plant-based protein for stir-fries, curries, and salads.

Grilled, baked, or sautéed for a meat substitute.

Blended into smoothies or used in desserts.

Benefits:

Plant-based protein source for muscle maintenance.

Low in saturated fats and cholesterol.

Contains essential amino acids and iron.

Protein Content:

Approximately 10 grams of protein per 3.5 ounces (firm, cooked).

Vitamin Composition:

Good source of B-vitamins like B1, B2, and B6.

Contains essential minerals like calcium, iron, and magnesium.

Low-calorie option, supporting weight management.

Calorie Count:

Low-calorie choice with approximately 144 calories per 3.5 ounces (firm, cooked).

Overall Impact on the Human Body:

Supports muscle health with plant-based protein.

Aids in maintaining a healthy weight with its low-calorie content.

Provides essential nutrients for overall well-being.

34. Lentils

Uses:

Cooked and added to salads, soups, stews, and curries.

Blended into dips, spreads, or vegetarian patties.

A versatile plant-based protein in various dishes.

Benefits:

High in fiber, promoting digestive health.

Rich in plant-based protein and essential amino acids.

Contains iron and folate for overall well-being.

Protein Content:

Approximately 9 grams of protein per 1/2 cup (cooked).

Vitamin Composition:

Good source of B-vitamins like folate and B6.

Contains essential minerals like iron, potassium, and manganese.

Low in calories, supporting weight management.

Calorie Count:

Nutrient-dense option with approximately 115 calories per 1/2 cup (cooked).

Overall Impact on the Human Body:

Supports digestive health and aids in weight management.

Provides plant-based protein and essential nutrients.

Contributes to overall well-being with its nutrient content.

35. Greek Yogurt

Uses:

Enjoyed on its own or with toppings like fruits and granola.

Used as a base for smoothies, dips, and salad dressings.

Added to desserts, baked goods, or frozen for a healthy treat.

Benefits:

High in protein, supporting muscle health.

Contains probiotics for gut health.

Rich in calcium and B-vitamins for overall well-being.

Protein Content:

Approximately 15 grams of protein per 6 ounces.

Vitamin Composition:

Excellent source of calcium and B-vitamins like B12 and riboflavin.

Contains essential minerals like phosphorus and potassium.

Low in calories, supporting weight management.

Chapter 8: Legumes

36. Chickpeas

Uses:

Cooked and added to salads, soups, and stews.

Blended into hummus or used in spreads and dips.

Roasted for a crunchy snack or added to trail mixes.

Benefits:

High in fiber, promoting digestive health.

Plant-based protein source for muscle maintenance.

Rich in essential nutrients like iron, folate, and manganese.

Protein Content:

Approximately 14.5 grams of protein per cup (cooked).

Vitamin Composition:

Good source of vitamins B6, folate, and C.

Contains essential minerals like iron, phosphorus, and zinc.

Supports heart health and aids in weight management.

Calorie Count:

Nutrient-dense option with approximately 269 calories per cup (cooked).

Overall Impact on the Human Body:

Supports digestive health with its high fiber content.

Provides plant-based protein and essential nutrients.

Contributes to heart health and helps regulate blood sugar.

37. Black Beans

Uses:

Cooked and added to burritos, tacos, and salads.

Blended into soups, stews, and chili.

Used in veggie burgers, dips, and casseroles.

Benefits:

High in fiber, promoting digestive health.

Plant-based protein source for muscle maintenance.

Rich in essential nutrients like iron, folate, and magnesium.

Protein Content:

Approximately 15.2 grams of protein per cup (cooked).

Vitamin Composition:

Good source of vitamins B1, B6, and folate.

Contains essential minerals like iron, phosphorus, and
potassium.

Supports heart health and aids in weight management.

Calorie Count:

Nutrient-dense option with approximately 227 calories per cup
(cooked).

Overall Impact on the Human Body:

Supports digestive health with its high fiber content.

Provides plant-based protein and essential nutrients.

Contributes to heart health and helps regulate blood sugar.

38. Red Lentils

Uses:

Cooked and added to curries, soups, and stews.

Blended into dips, spreads, and sauces.

Used in salads, casseroles, and veggie patties.

Benefits:

High in fiber, promoting digestive health.

Plant-based protein source for muscle maintenance.

Rich in essential nutrients like iron, folate, and manganese.

Protein Content:

Approximately 17.9 grams of protein per cup (cooked).

Vitamin Composition:

Good source of vitamins B1, B6, and folate.

Contains essential minerals like iron, phosphorus, and potassium.

Supports heart health and aids in weight management.

Calorie Count:

Nutrient-dense option with approximately 230 calories per cup (cooked).

Overall Impact on the Human Body:

Supports digestive health with its high fiber content.

Provides plant-based protein and essential nutrients.

Contributes to heart health and helps regulate blood sugar.

39. Pinto Beans

Uses:

Cooked and added to burritos, chili, and salads.

Blended into dips, spreads, and refried beans.

Used in casseroles, soups, and veggie burgers.

Benefits:

High in fiber, promoting digestive health.

Plant-based protein source for muscle maintenance.

Rich in essential nutrients like iron, folate, and manganese.

Protein Content:

Approximately 15.4 grams of protein per cup (cooked).

Vitamin Composition:

Good source of vitamins B1, B6, and folate.

Contains essential minerals like iron, phosphorus, and potassium.

Supports heart health and aids in weight management.

Calorie Count:

Nutrient-dense option with approximately 245 calories per cup (cooked).

Overall Impact on the Human Body:

Supports digestive health with its high fiber content.

Provides plant-based protein and essential nutrients.

Contributes to heart health and helps regulate blood sugar.

40. Kidney Beans

Uses:

Cooked and added to chili, salads, and casseroles.

Blended into dips, spreads, and veggie burgers.

Used in soups, stews, and rice dishes.

Benefits:

High in fiber, promoting digestive health.

Plant-based protein source for muscle maintenance.

Rich in essential nutrients like iron, folate, and manganese.

Protein Content:

Approximately 15.3 grams of protein per cup (cooked).

Vitamin Composition:

Good source of vitamins B1, B6, and folate.

Contains essential minerals like iron, phosphorus, and potassium.

Supports heart health and aids in weight management.

Calorie Count:

Nutrient-dense option with approximately 225 calories per cup (cooked).

Overall Impact on the Human Body:

Supports digestive health with its high fiber content.

Provides plant-based protein and essential nutrients.

Contributes to heart health and helps regulate blood sugar.

Chapter 9: Cruciferous Vegetables

41. Broccoli

Uses:

Steamed or roasted as a side dish.

Added to salads, stir-fries, and casseroles.

Blended into soups or enjoyed raw with dip.

Benefits:

High in fiber, promoting digestive health.

Rich in vitamins C and K, supporting immune and bone health.

Contains sulforaphane, which may have anti-cancer properties.

Protein Content:

Approximately 2.6 grams of protein per cup (cooked).

Vitamin Composition:

Excellent source of vitamins C and K.

Contains B-vitamins like folate and vitamin B6.

Provides essential minerals like potassium and manganese.

Calorie Count:

Low-calorie option with approximately 55 calories per cup (cooked).

Overall Impact on the Human Body:

Supports immune and bone health with its rich nutrient content.

May have anti-cancer properties due to sulforaphane.

Contributes to heart health and aids in weight management.

42. Cauliflower

Uses:

Roasted or mashed as a low-carb alternative.

Added to salads, soups, and casseroles.

Blended into sauces, such as cauliflower Alfredo.

Benefits:

High in fiber, promoting digestive health.

Rich in vitamins C and K, supporting immune and bone health.

Contains choline, essential for brain health and development.

Protein Content:

Approximately 2.0 grams of protein per cup (cooked).

Vitamin Composition:

Excellent source of vitamins C and K.

Contains B-vitamins like folate and vitamin B6.

Provides essential minerals like potassium and manganese.

Calorie Count:

Low-calorie option with approximately 29 calories per cup (cooked).

Overall Impact on the Human Body:

Supports immune and bone health with its rich nutrient content.

Contributes to brain health and development with choline.

Aids in weight management as a low-calorie alternative.

43. Brussels Sprouts

Uses:

Roasted, sautéed, or steamed as a side dish.

Added to salads, stir-fries, and casseroles.

Shredded and used in slaws or as a topping for pizzas.

Benefits:

High in fiber, promoting digestive health.

Rich in vitamins C and K, supporting immune and bone health.

Contains antioxidants, reducing oxidative stress.

Protein Content:

Approximately 3.0 grams of protein per cup (cooked).

Vitamin Composition:

Excellent source of vitamins C and K.

Contains B-vitamins like folate and vitamin B6.

Provides essential minerals like potassium and manganese.

Calorie Count:

Low-calorie option with approximately 56 calories per cup (cooked).

Overall Impact on the Human Body:

Supports immune and bone health with its rich nutrient content.

Contributes to heart health and aids in weight management.

Provides antioxidants, reducing oxidative stress.

44. Kale

Uses:

Added to salads, smoothies, and wraps.

Sautéed, baked, or added to soups and stews.

Used as a base for kale chips or in pesto.

Benefits:

High in fiber, promoting digestive health.

Rich in vitamins A, C, and K, supporting immune and bone health.

Contains antioxidants, reducing oxidative stress.

Protein Content:

Approximately 2.9 grams of protein per cup (cooked).

Vitamin Composition:

Excellent source of vitamins A, C, and K.

Contains B-vitamins like folate and vitamin B6.

Provides essential minerals like potassium and manganese.

Calorie Count:

Low-calorie option with approximately 33 calories per cup (cooked).

Overall Impact on the Human Body:

Supports immune and bone health with its rich nutrient content.

Contributes to heart health and aids in weight management.

Provides antioxidants, reducing oxidative stress.

45. Cabbage

Uses:

Shredded and added to slaws, salads, and wraps.

Used in stir-fries, soups, and stews.

Fermented into sauerkraut for gut health.

Benefits:

High in fiber, promoting digestive health.

Rich in vitamins C and K, supporting immune and bone health.

Contains antioxidants, reducing oxidative stress.

Protein Content:

Approximately 1.3 grams of protein per cup (cooked).

Vitamin Composition:

Excellent source of vitamins C and K.

Contains B-vitamins like folate and vitamin B6.

Provides essential minerals like potassium and manganese.

Calorie Count:

Low-calorie option with approximately 22 calories per cup (cooked).

Overall Impact on the Human Body:

Supports immune and bone health with its rich nutrient content.

Contributes to heart health and aids in weight management.

Provides antioxidants, reducing oxidative stress.

Chapter 10: Berries

46. Blueberries

Uses:

Added to cereals, yogurt, and smoothie bowls.

Used in baking, such as muffins, pancakes, and desserts.

Enjoyed as a snack on their own or mixed with other fruits.

Benefits:

High in antioxidants, reducing oxidative stress.

Rich in vitamins C and K, supporting immune and bone health.

Contains anthocyanins, which may have anti-inflammatory properties.

Protein Content:

Approximately 0.7 grams of protein per cup.

Vitamin Composition:

Excellent source of vitamins C and K.

Contains B-vitamins like folate and vitamin B6.

Provides essential minerals like manganese and potassium.

Calorie Count:

Low-calorie option with approximately 84 calories per cup.

Overall Impact on the Human Body:

Provides antioxidants, reducing oxidative stress.

Supports immune and bone health with its rich nutrient content.

May have anti-inflammatory properties due to anthocyanins.

47. Strawberries

Uses:

Sliced and added to cereals, salads, and desserts.

Blended into smoothies, sauces, and jams.

Enjoyed as a fresh snack or dipped in dark chocolate.

Benefits:

High in antioxidants, reducing oxidative stress.

Rich in vitamin C, supporting immune health and collagen production.

Contains manganese, essential for bone health.

Protein Content:

Approximately 1.0 gram of protein per cup.

Vitamin Composition:

Excellent source of vitamin C.

Contains B-vitamins like folate and vitamin B6.

Provides essential minerals like manganese and potassium.

Calorie Count:

Low-calorie option with approximately 50 calories per cup.

Overall Impact on the Human Body:

Provides antioxidants, reducing oxidative stress.

Supports immune health and collagen production with vitamin C.

Contributes to bone health with manganese.

48. Raspberries

Uses:

Added to cereals, yogurt, and desserts.

Blended into smoothies, sauces, and sorbets.

Enjoyed as a fresh snack or paired with cheese.

Benefits:

High in antioxidants, reducing oxidative stress.

Rich in fiber, promoting digestive health.

Contains vitamin C and manganese for overall well-being.

Protein Content:

Approximately 1.5 grams of protein per cup.

Vitamin Composition:

Excellent source of vitamin C.

Contains B-vitamins like folate and vitamin B6.

Provides essential minerals like manganese and potassium.

Calorie Count:

Low-calorie option with approximately 65 calories per cup.

Overall Impact on the Human Body:

Provides antioxidants, reducing oxidative stress.

Supports digestive health with its high fiber content.

Contributes to overall well-being with vitamin C and manganese.

49. Blackberries

Uses:

Added to cereals, salads, and desserts.

Blended into smoothies, sauces, and jams.

Enjoyed as a fresh snack or added to savory dishes.

Benefits:

High in antioxidants, reducing oxidative stress.

Rich in fiber, promoting digestive health.

Contains vitamin C and manganese for overall well-being.

Protein Content:

Approximately 2.0 grams of protein per cup.

Vitamin Composition:

Excellent source of vitamin C.

Contains B-vitamins like folate and vitamin B6.

Provides essential minerals like manganese and potassium.

Calorie Count:

Low-calorie option with approximately 62 calories per cup.

Overall Impact on the Human Body:

Provides antioxidants, reducing oxidative stress.

Supports digestive health with its high fiber content.

Contributes to overall well-being with vitamin C and manganese.

50. Cranberries

Uses:

Added to cereals, salads, and desserts.

Used in sauces, relishes, and chutneys.

Enjoyed as a fresh snack or dried in trail mixes.

Benefits:

High in antioxidants, reducing oxidative stress.

Contains proanthocyanidins, which may support urinary tract health.

Provides vitamin C and manganese for overall well-being.

Protein Content:

Approximately 0.4 grams of protein per cup.

Vitamin Composition:

Good source of vitamin C.

Contains B-vitamins like folate and vitamin B6.

Provides essential minerals like manganese and potassium.

Calorie Count:

Low-calorie option with approximately 51 calories per cup.

Overall Impact on the Human Body:

Provides antioxidants, reducing oxidative stress.

May support urinary tract health with proanthocyanidins.

Contributes to overall well-being with vitamin C and manganese.

www.ingramcontent.com/pod-product-compliance
Lightning Source LLC
Chambersburg PA
CBHW070822280726
48660CB00017B/2422